DR. BARBARA 7-DAY CANCER CURE

Discover Dr. Barbara's proven 7-days cancer cure.
Transformative insight and strategies for rapid healing.
Empower yourself with life-changing solution for fighting
cancer naturally and effectively

Miguel Sofia

Table of Contents

COPYRIGHT © 2023

CHAPTER ONE

Introduction to Dr. Barbara's Holistic Approach to Cancer Healing

In the realm of cancer treatment, Dr. Barbara's holistic approach stands out as a beacon of comprehensive care. Rooted in the understanding that cancer affects not only the physical body but also the mind, emotions, and spirit, Dr. Barbara's methodology encompasses a wide range of modalities aimed at addressing the entirety of the individual. Unlike conventional cancer treatments that often focus solely on eradicating tumors through surgery, chemotherapy, and radiation, Dr. Barbara's approach recognizes the interconnectedness of all aspects of health and seeks to promote healing on multiple levels simultaneously.

Understanding Holistic Healing

At the core of Dr. Barbara's approach is the concept of holistic healing. Holistic health is a philosophy that views the body, mind, and spirit as interconnected and seeks to address imbalances in all areas to promote overall well-being. Rather than simply treating symptoms or isolated parts of the body, holistic healing aims to restore harmony and balance to the entire individual. This approach acknowledges that physical ailments can be influenced by emotional, mental, and spiritual factors, and therefore requires a comprehensive treatment plan that addresses all aspects of a person's health.

The Role of Conventional Medicine

While Dr. Barbara's holistic approach emphasizes alternative and complementary therapies, it does not dismiss the importance of conventional medicine in cancer treatment. Instead, it seeks to integrate the best of both worlds to provide patients with the most effective and well-rounded care possible. Conventional treatments such as surgery, chemotherapy, and radiation may be utilized when necessary to target and eliminate cancerous cells. However, these treatments are often supplemented with holistic therapies to support the body's natural healing processes, minimize side effects, and promote overall health and well-being.

Nutritional Healing

One cornerstone of Dr. Barbara's holistic approach is nutritional healing. Food is viewed not only as fuel for the body but also as medicine that can nourish and heal. A diet rich in whole, nutrient-dense foods such as fruits, vegetables, whole grains, and lean proteins forms the foundation of Dr. Barbara's nutritional approach. These foods provide essential vitamins, minerals, antioxidants, and other nutrients that support immune function, reduce inflammation, and promote cellular health. In addition to emphasizing healthy eating, Dr. Barbara may also recommend specific dietary supplements or herbal remedies to address individual needs and support the body's healing process.

Mind-Body Medicine

Another integral component of Dr. Barbara's holistic approach is mind-body medicine. This approach recognizes the powerful connection between the mind and body and seeks to harness the body's innate healing abilities through techniques such as meditation, visualization, breathwork, and relaxation exercises. These practices not only help to reduce stress and anxiety but also promote a sense of empowerment and control over one's health. By cultivating a positive mindset and tapping into the body's natural healing resources, patients can enhance their overall well-being and support their recovery from cancer.

Emotional and Spiritual Support

In addition to addressing the physical and mental aspects of health, Dr. Barbara's holistic approach also places great importance on emotional and spiritual support. A cancer diagnosis can be emotionally devastating, and it's essential for patients to have outlets for processing their feelings and finding meaning and purpose in their journey. Dr. Barbara may recommend therapies such as counseling, support groups, art therapy, or spiritual practices to help patients navigate the emotional and existential challenges of cancer. By addressing the deeper emotional and spiritual dimensions of healing, patients can experience greater peace, resilience, and inner strength.

Complementary Therapies

Complementary therapies play a significant role in Dr. Barbara's holistic approach to cancer healing. These therapies work alongside conventional treatments to enhance their effectiveness, reduce side effects, and improve overall quality of life. Examples of complementary therapies commonly used in Dr. Barbara's practice include acupuncture, massage therapy, yoga, tai chi, energy healing, and aromatherapy. These modalities help to support the body's natural healing mechanisms, alleviate pain and discomfort, and promote relaxation and well-being. By integrating a variety of complementary therapies into the treatment plan, patients can experience holistic healing on multiple levels.

Personalized Treatment Plans

Central to Dr. Barbara's holistic approach is the recognition that each individual is unique and requires personalized care tailored to their specific needs and circumstances. Rather than taking a one-size-fits-all approach, Dr. Barbara works closely with each patient to develop a comprehensive treatment plan that addresses their physical, emotional, mental, and spiritual health. This may involve a combination of conventional treatments, nutritional interventions, mind-body practices, complementary therapies, and emotional support strategies customized to meet the individual's needs and preferences. By treating the whole person rather than just the disease, Dr. Barbara empowers patients to take an active role in their healing journey and optimize their chances of recovery and long-term wellness.

Conclusion

In conclusion, Dr. Barbara's holistic approach to cancer healing offers a comprehensive and integrated model of care that addresses the physical, emotional, mental, and spiritual aspects of health. By recognizing the interconnectedness of all aspects of a person's well-being and incorporating a variety of modalities from both conventional and alternative medicine, Dr. Barbara provides patients with a holistic treatment plan that supports their body's natural healing processes and promotes overall wellness. Through personalized care, compassionate support, and a commitment to treating the whole person, Dr. Barbara empowers patients to embark on a journey of healing, resilience, and transformation in the face of cancer.

CHAPTER TWO

Understanding Cancer: Dr. Barbara's Insights into the Disease

Cancer, a complex and multifaceted disease, has been a subject of intensive research and exploration for centuries. Dr. Barbara, with her comprehensive understanding and holistic approach to healthcare, provides profound insights into the nature of cancer. Through her work, she sheds light on the underlying mechanisms of cancer development, the factors influencing its progression, and the holistic strategies for prevention and treatment.

The Nature of Cancer

Cancer is characterized by the uncontrolled growth and spread of abnormal cells in the body. These cells, which can originate from any tissue or organ, divide and proliferate rapidly, forming tumors and invading surrounding tissues. Unlike normal cells, cancer cells lack the mechanisms that regulate growth and apoptosis (programmed cell death), allowing them to accumulate and proliferate unchecked. Over time, cancer cells can metastasize, spreading to distant parts of the body and causing further damage.

Dr. Barbara emphasizes the importance of understanding cancer at the molecular level. Advances in molecular biology have revealed the intricate molecular mechanisms underlying cancer development, including mutations in oncogenes (genes that promote cell growth) and tumor suppressor genes (genes that inhibit cell growth), dysregulation of signaling pathways, and alterations in the tumor microenvironment. By unraveling the molecular intricacies of cancer, researchers and clinicians can identify novel therapeutic targets and develop more effective treatments.

Risk Factors and Prevention

While the exact causes of cancer are complex and multifactorial, certain risk factors have been identified that increase an individual's likelihood of developing the disease. These risk factors may include genetic predisposition, environmental exposures (such as tobacco smoke, UV radiation, and carcinogenic chemicals), lifestyle factors (such as diet, physical activity, and alcohol consumption), and infectious agents (such as human papillomavirus and Helicobacter pylori).

Dr. Barbara emphasizes the importance of cancer prevention through lifestyle modifications and risk reduction strategies. By adopting a healthy lifestyle that includes a balanced diet, regular exercise, avoidance of tobacco and excessive alcohol consumption, and sun protection, individuals can reduce their risk of developing cancer. Additionally, early detection through regular screenings and awareness of warning signs can lead to earlier diagnosis and more favorable treatment outcomes.

Holistic Approaches to Cancer Treatment

In treating cancer, Dr. Barbara advocates for a holistic approach that addresses the whole person, not just the disease. Conventional treatments such as surgery, chemotherapy, and radiation may be necessary to target and eliminate cancerous cells. However, these treatments are often accompanied by significant side effects and can take a toll on the body and mind.

Dr. Barbara emphasizes the importance of integrating complementary and alternative therapies into cancer treatment plans to support the body's natural healing processes, alleviate side effects, and improve quality of life. These therapies may include nutritional interventions, mind-body practices (such as meditation, yoga, and acupuncture), botanical medicine, energy healing, and emotional support services. By combining conventional and holistic modalities, patients can experience more comprehensive care that addresses their physical, emotional, mental, and spiritual needs.

The Role of the Immune System

The immune system plays a crucial role in cancer surveillance and defense. Under normal circumstances, the immune system can recognize and eliminate abnormal cells before they have a chance to develop into cancer. However, cancer cells can evade immune detection and suppression, allowing tumors to proliferate and metastasize.

Dr. Barbara highlights the emerging field of immunotherapy, which harnesses the power of the immune system to target and destroy cancer cells. Immunotherapy includes various approaches such as immune checkpoint inhibitors, adoptive cell therapy, and cancer vaccines, which enhance the body's immune response against cancer. By unleashing the immune system's potential to recognize and eradicate cancer cells, immunotherapy offers promising new avenues for cancer treatment.

Conclusion

In conclusion, Dr. Barbara's insights into cancer provide a comprehensive understanding of the disease, its risk factors, and its treatment options. By recognizing cancer as a complex interplay of genetic, environmental, and lifestyle factors, Dr. Barbara underscores the importance of holistic approaches to prevention and treatment. Through a combination of conventional therapies, complementary modalities, and immunotherapy, patients can receive comprehensive care that addresses their physical, emotional, and spiritual needs, empowering them to overcome cancer and thrive.

CHAPTER THREE

The Role of Herbs in Cancer Treatment: Exploring Their Therapeutic Potential

Herbal medicine has been utilized for centuries in the treatment of various ailments, including cancer. Dr. Barbara, with her holistic approach to healthcare, recognizes the therapeutic potential of herbs in cancer treatment. By exploring the mechanisms of action, evidence-based research, and clinical applications of herbs, Dr. Barbara sheds light on their role in supporting conventional cancer therapies and promoting overall well-being.

Historical Context and Traditional Use

Herbal medicine has a rich and diverse history that spans cultures and civilizations around the world. Traditional healers and herbalists have long relied on the medicinal properties of plants to treat a wide range of illnesses, including cancer. Ancient texts and traditional systems of medicine, such as Traditional Chinese Medicine (TCM), Ayurveda, and Native American healing practices, document the use of specific herbs and botanical remedies for cancer prevention and treatment.

Dr. Barbara emphasizes the importance of respecting traditional wisdom and cultural practices when exploring the role of herbs in cancer treatment. While modern scientific research has provided valuable insights into the therapeutic properties of herbs, it is essential to integrate this knowledge with traditional knowledge and holistic approaches to healthcare.

Mechanisms of Action

Herbs contain a diverse array of bioactive compounds that exert therapeutic effects on the body. Many herbs possess anti-inflammatory, antioxidant, immunomodulatory, and anti-cancer properties that can target various stages of cancer development and progression. Some herbs may inhibit tumor growth by inducing apoptosis (programmed cell death) in cancer cells, blocking angiogenesis (the formation of new blood vessels to supply tumors), or enhancing the immune system's ability to recognize and destroy cancer cells.

Dr. Barbara highlights the importance of understanding the mechanisms of action of herbs in cancer treatment. By elucidating the molecular pathways and biological processes involved, researchers can identify potential targets for drug development and optimize the use of herbal remedies in cancer therapy.

Evidence-Based Research

While traditional knowledge provides valuable insights into the potential therapeutic benefits of herbs, modern scientific research plays a critical role in validating their efficacy and safety. Numerous studies have investigated the anti-cancer properties of various herbs and botanical compounds, both in vitro (in laboratory studies) and in vivo (in animal studies and clinical trials).

Dr. Barbara emphasizes the importance of evidence-based research in evaluating the efficacy of herbs in cancer treatment. Rigorous scientific studies, including randomized controlled trials (RCTs) and meta-analyses, provide valuable data on the safety, efficacy, and optimal dosing of herbal remedies. By integrating high-quality research into clinical practice, healthcare providers can make informed decisions about the use of herbs in cancer therapy and ensure the highest standards of patient care.

Commonly Used Herbs in Cancer Treatment

A wide variety of herbs and botanical remedies have been studied for their potential anti-cancer properties. Some of the most commonly used herbs in cancer treatment include:

- **Turmeric (Curcuma longa)**: Known for its anti-inflammatory and antioxidant properties, turmeric contains the active compound curcumin, which has been shown to inhibit tumor growth and metastasis in various types of cancer.

- **Green Tea (Camellia sinensis)**: Rich in polyphenols and catechins, green tea has been studied for its potential anti-cancer effects. Epidemiological studies have suggested that regular consumption of green tea may lower the risk of certain cancers, including breast, prostate, and colorectal cancer.

- **Ginger (Zingiber officinale)**: Ginger contains bioactive compounds such as gingerol and shogaol, which exhibit anti-inflammatory and anti-cancer properties. Studies have shown that ginger extract may inhibit the growth and spread of cancer cells in vitro and in animal models.

- **Garlic (Allium sativum)**: Garlic is rich in organosulfur compounds, which have been shown to possess anti-cancer effects. Population studies have suggested that higher garlic consumption may be associated with a reduced risk of certain cancers, including stomach and colorectal cancer.

- **Mushrooms (Various species)**: Certain medicinal mushrooms, such as reishi (Ganoderma lucidum), shiitake (Lentinula edodes), and maitake (Grifolafrondosa), contain bioactive compounds that may stimulate the immune system and inhibit tumor growth.

Dr. Barbara emphasizes the importance of individualized treatment plans that take into account the specific needs and preferences of each patient. While herbs may offer valuable therapeutic benefits, it is essential to consult with a qualified healthcare provider knowledgeable in herbal medicine to ensure safe and effective use.

Integration with Conventional Cancer Therapies

Incorporating herbs into conventional cancer treatment plans requires careful consideration and coordination with healthcare providers. Herbs have the potential to interact with certain medications and treatments, so it is essential to discuss their use with a qualified healthcare professional.

Dr. Barbara emphasizes the importance of an integrative approach to cancer treatment that combines the best of conventional and complementary therapies. Herbs may complement conventional treatments such as surgery, chemotherapy, and radiation by enhancing their efficacy, reducing side effects, and supporting the body's natural healing processes.

Conclusion

In conclusion, herbs play a significant role in cancer treatment, offering a natural and holistic approach to supporting health and well-being. Dr. Barbara's insights into the therapeutic potential of herbs provide valuable guidance for patients and healthcare providers seeking comprehensive and personalized cancer care. By understanding the mechanisms of action, evidence-based research, and clinical applications of herbs, individuals can make informed decisions about their use in cancer treatment and promote optimal outcomes for cancer patients.

CHAPTER FOUR

Preparing for Your Healing Journey: Mental and Physical Readiness for the 7-Day Program

Embarking on a healing journey, especially one as intensive as a 7-day program, requires careful preparation both mentally and physically. Dr. Barbara's holistic approach to health and wellness emphasizes the importance of addressing the whole person—mind, body, and spirit—in order to achieve optimal healing outcomes. By taking proactive steps to prepare yourself mentally and physically for the journey ahead, you can maximize the benefits of the program and set yourself up for success.

Understanding the Program

Before diving into the preparation process, it's essential to have a clear understanding of the 7-day program you'll be participating in. Familiarize yourself with the program's goals, structure, and activities so that you know what to expect during each day of the program. Take the time to review any materials provided by the program organizers, such as schedules, dietary guidelines, and recommended activities.

Setting Intentions

Setting intentions for your healing journey can help to focus your mind and clarify your goals for the program. Take some time to reflect on what you hope to achieve during the 7-day program, whether it's physical healing, emotional release, spiritual growth, or simply a renewed sense of well-being. Write down your intentions and revisit them regularly throughout the program to stay aligned with your goals.

Mental Preparation

Preparing yourself mentally for the 7-day program involves cultivating a positive mindset and an open attitude towards healing and transformation. Practice mindfulness techniques such as meditation, deep breathing, or visualization to calm the mind and reduce stress and anxiety. Cultivate an attitude of curiosity, receptivity, and non-judgment towards whatever experiences may arise during the program, knowing that each moment holds the potential for growth and healing.

Physical Preparation

In addition to mental preparation, it's important to ensure that your body is physically ready for the demands of the 7-day program. Pay attention to your diet, hydration, and sleep in the days leading up to the program to support your overall health and well-being. Eat a balanced diet rich in whole foods, fruits, vegetables, and lean proteins, and stay hydrated by drinking plenty of water throughout the day. Aim to get adequate restorative sleep each night to recharge your body and mind for the challenges ahead.

Detoxification

Many healing programs incorporate detoxification protocols to cleanse the body of toxins and impurities that may be hindering the healing process. If your 7-day program includes detoxification elements such as fasting, juicing, or cleansing diets, it's important to prepare your body accordingly. Gradually reduce your intake of caffeine, sugar, processed foods, and alcohol in the days leading up to the program to minimize withdrawal symptoms and support the detoxification process.

Gathering Supplies

Depending on the specific requirements of the 7-day program, you may need to gather supplies or equipment to support your participation. This could include yoga mats, meditation cushions, journaling supplies, herbal supplements, or any other materials recommended by the program organizers. Take the time to gather everything you'll need in advance so that you can fully immerse yourself in the program without interruption.

Support System

Lastly, consider enlisting the support of friends, family members, or fellow participants to accompany you on your healing journey. Having a supportive network of people who understand and respect your commitment to healing can provide invaluable encouragement, accountability, and companionship throughout the program. Share your intentions and goals with your support system and lean on them for guidance and encouragement when needed.

Conclusion

Preparing for a 7-day healing program requires a holistic approach that addresses both mental and physical readiness. By setting clear intentions, cultivating a positive mindset, supporting your body with nourishing food and rest, and gathering necessary supplies, you can ensure that you're fully prepared to embark on your healing journey. With dedication, openness, and support, you can maximize the benefits of the program and experience profound transformation and healing on all levels—mind, body, and spirit.

CHAPTER FIVE

Day 1: Initiating Your Cancer Cure with Herbal Remedies and Nutrient-Dense Foods

Day 1 marks the beginning of your journey towards healing and wellness, focusing on the integration of herbal remedies and nutrient-dense foods into your daily routine. Dr. Barbara's holistic approach emphasizes the importance of utilizing the healing properties of herbs and nourishing your body with wholesome, nutrient-rich foods to support your immune system, promote cellular health, and initiate your path towards cancer cure.

Herbal Remedies

Herbal remedies have been used for centuries in traditional medicine systems around the world to support health and treat various ailments, including cancer. Today, modern research continues to uncover the therapeutic potential of herbs in cancer prevention and treatment. On Day 1 of your healing journey, you'll have the opportunity to explore a variety of herbal remedies carefully selected to support your body's natural healing processes.

Dr. Barbara recommends incorporating a range of cancer-fighting herbs into your daily routine, such as turmeric, ginger, garlic, green tea, and medicinal mushrooms. These herbs contain bioactive compounds with anti-inflammatory, antioxidant, and anti-cancer properties that can help to inhibit tumor growth, support immune function, and reduce inflammation in the body. Whether consumed as teas, tinctures, supplements, or added to meals, these herbal remedies can complement your overall cancer treatment plan and promote your journey towards healing.

Nutrient-Dense Foods

Nutrition plays a crucial role in supporting overall health and well-being, especially during cancer treatment. Nutrient-dense foods provide essential vitamins, minerals, antioxidants, and phytonutrients that support immune function, promote cellular health, and optimize your body's ability to heal. On Day 1, you'll have the opportunity to nourish your body with a variety of nutrient-dense foods carefully selected to support your cancer cure journey.

Dr. Barbara recommends focusing on whole, minimally processed foods that are rich in nutrients and free from artificial additives and preservatives. Incorporate plenty of fresh fruits and vegetables, whole grains, legumes, nuts, seeds, and lean proteins into your meals to provide your body with the essential building blocks it needs for optimal health and healing. Aim to consume a rainbow of colors to ensure a diverse array of nutrients and phytochemicals, and prioritize organic and locally sourced foods whenever possible to minimize exposure to pesticides and other harmful chemicals.

Meal Planning and Preparation

Effective meal planning and preparation are essential for success on Day 1 and throughout your healing journey. Take the time to plan out your meals and snacks for the day, ensuring that they are balanced, nutritious, and aligned with your dietary preferences and goals. Batch cook and pre-portion meals and snacks to make healthy eating more convenient and accessible, especially during busy days or times when you may be feeling fatigued.

Dr. Barbara recommends incorporating a variety of cancer-fighting foods into your meals and snacks, such as leafy greens, cruciferous vegetables, berries, citrus fruits, whole grains, beans, lentils, nuts, and seeds. Experiment with different cooking methods and flavor combinations to keep your meals interesting and enjoyable, and don't forget to stay hydrated by drinking plenty of water throughout the day.

Mindful Eating and Gratitude

As you nourish your body with herbal remedies and nutrient-dense foods on Day 1, remember to practice mindful eating and cultivate gratitude for the abundance of nourishment and healing that you are receiving. Take the time to savor each bite, paying attention to the flavors, textures, and sensations of the food, and listen to your body's hunger and fullness cues. Express gratitude for the farmers, producers, and caregivers who have contributed to the food on your plate, and for the opportunity to support your body's healing journey through conscious nutrition.

By incorporating herbal remedies and nutrient-dense foods into your daily routine on Day 1, you are taking an important step towards initiating your cancer cure journey. Embrace the healing power of nature's pharmacy and the nourishment of wholesome foods as you embark on this transformative path towards health and wellness.

CHAPTER SIX

Days 2-3: Deepening the Healing Process with Specific Herbal Formulas and Teas

As you progress through your healing journey, Days 2 and 3 offer an opportunity to deepen the healing process by incorporating specific herbal formulas and teas into your daily routine. Dr. Barbara's holistic approach emphasizes the synergistic effects of combining targeted herbal remedies with mindful consumption of herbal teas to support your body's natural healing processes and promote overall well-being.

Herbal Formulas

On Days 2 and 3, you'll have the opportunity to explore specific herbal formulas carefully selected to address your individual health needs and support your healing journey. These herbal formulas may include combinations of herbs known for their synergistic effects on specific health conditions, such as immune support, detoxification, inflammation reduction, or stress relief.

Dr. Barbara recommends consulting with a qualified herbalist or healthcare provider to identify the most appropriate herbal formulas for your unique health concerns and goals. These formulas may be available in various forms, including tinctures, capsules, powders, or extracts, and can be taken according to the recommended dosage instructions to maximize their therapeutic benefits.

Herbal Teas

In addition to herbal formulas, herbal teas offer a convenient and enjoyable way to incorporate the healing properties of herbs into your daily routine. Herbal teas are made by steeping dried herbs in hot water, allowing their medicinal compounds to infuse into the liquid for a soothing and therapeutic beverage.

Dr. Barbara recommends exploring a variety of herbal teas known for their health-promoting properties, such as chamomile, peppermint, ginger, dandelion root, and echinacea. These teas can be enjoyed throughout the day as a refreshing alternative to water or other beverages, providing hydration and a gentle boost to your body's natural healing processes.

Mindful Consumption

As you incorporate specific herbal formulas and teas into your daily routine on Days 2 and 3, remember to practice mindful consumption and pay attention to how your body responds to the herbs. Notice any changes in your energy levels, mood, digestion, or overall sense of well-being, and adjust your herbal regimen accordingly to optimize your healing experience.

Dr. Barbara emphasizes the importance of listening to your body's signals and honoring its needs as you navigate your healing journey. If you experience any adverse reactions or discomfort from a particular herb or formula, discontinue use and consult with a healthcare professional for guidance. Similarly, if you find that certain herbs resonate more strongly with you and provide noticeable benefits, consider incorporating them more frequently into your daily routine.

Self-Care Practices

In addition to herbal remedies and teas, Days 2 and 3 offer an opportunity to deepen the healing process through self-care practices that nourish your body, mind, and spirit. Take time each day to engage in activities that promote relaxation, stress reduction, and emotional well-being, such as meditation, deep breathing, gentle exercise, journaling, or spending time in nature.

Dr. Barbara encourages you to prioritize self-care and make time for activities that bring you joy, peace, and inner harmony. By nurturing yourself on all levels—physically, mentally, emotionally, and spiritually—you can create an optimal environment for healing to occur and support your body's innate ability to restore balance and vitality.

Conclusion

Days 2 and 3 of your healing journey offer an opportunity to deepen the healing process with specific herbal formulas and teas designed to support your individual health needs and goals. By incorporating targeted herbal remedies into your daily routine and practicing mindful consumption, you can enhance the therapeutic benefits of herbs and promote overall well-being. Additionally, prioritize self-care practices that nurture your body, mind, and spirit, creating an optimal environment for healing to occur. With dedication, mindfulness, and a commitment to holistic wellness, you can continue to progress on your journey towards health, vitality, and wholeness.

CHAPTER SEVEN

Days 4-5: Supporting Your Body's Natural Defenses with Herbal Tonics and Supplements

As you move forward on your healing journey, Days 4 and 5 present an opportunity to further support your body's natural defenses and promote overall wellness through the use of herbal tonics and supplements. Dr. Barbara's holistic approach emphasizes the importance of nourishing the body with targeted herbal formulations and nutritional supplements to optimize immune function, enhance vitality, and facilitate the healing process.

Herbal Tonics

Herbal tonics are concentrated liquid preparations made from a combination of herbs known for their tonic and adaptogenic properties. These herbal formulations are designed to support overall health and vitality by promoting balance and resilience in the body's systems. On Days 4 and 5, you'll have the opportunity to incorporate herbal tonics into your daily routine to nourish your body from the inside out.

Dr. Barbara recommends exploring a variety of herbal tonics that target specific areas of health and well-being, such as immune support, stress relief, energy enhancement, or hormonal balance. These tonics may contain a blend of adaptogenic herbs, immune-boosting botanicals, and nourishing plant extracts that work synergistically to promote resilience and vitality. Take these tonics according to the recommended dosage instructions to maximize their therapeutic benefits and support your body's natural defenses.

Nutritional Supplements

In addition to herbal tonics, nutritional supplements offer a convenient and effective way to enhance your body's nutrient intake and support optimal health and wellness. On Days 4 and 5, you'll have the opportunity to explore a variety of supplements that target specific nutritional deficiencies or health concerns, such as vitamin and mineral supplements, omega-3 fatty acids, probiotics, and antioxidants.

Dr. Barbara recommends consulting with a qualified healthcare provider or nutritionist to identify the most appropriate supplements for your individual needs and goals. These supplements can help to fill nutrient gaps in your diet, support immune function, and optimize your body's ability to heal and thrive. Take these supplements as directed, paying attention to any specific instructions or precautions provided by your healthcare provider.

Hydration and Rest

As you incorporate herbal tonics and supplements into your daily routine on Days 4 and 5, remember to prioritize hydration and rest to support your body's healing process. Drink plenty of water throughout the day to stay hydrated and facilitate the elimination of toxins from your body. Adequate hydration is essential for maintaining optimal cellular function, supporting digestion, and promoting overall well-being.

Similarly, prioritize rest and relaxation to allow your body time to repair, regenerate, and recharge. Aim for at least 7-8 hours of restorative sleep each night to support your body's natural healing processes and promote overall vitality. Take breaks throughout the day to rest and recharge, engaging in activities that promote relaxation and stress reduction, such as meditation, deep breathing, or gentle movement.

Mindful Awareness

As you support your body's natural defenses with herbal tonics and supplements on Days 4 and 5, cultivate mindful awareness of how your body responds to these interventions. Notice any changes in your energy levels, mood, digestion, or overall sense of well-being, and adjust your regimen accordingly to optimize your healing experience.

Dr. Barbara encourages you to listen to your body's signals and honor its needs as you navigate your healing journey. If you experience any adverse reactions or discomfort from a particular tonic or supplement, discontinue use and consult with a healthcare professional for guidance. Similarly, if you find that certain tonics or supplements resonate more strongly with you and provide noticeable benefits, consider incorporating them more frequently into your daily routine.

Conclusion

Days 4 and 5 of your healing journey offer an opportunity to support your body's natural defenses and promote overall wellness through the use of herbal tonics and supplements. By nourishing your body with targeted herbal formulations and nutritional supplements, hydrating adequately, prioritizing rest and relaxation, and cultivating mindful awareness, you can create an optimal environment for healing to occur. With dedication, mindfulness, and a commitment to holistic wellness, you can continue to progress on your journey towards health, vitality, and wholeness.

CHAPTER EIGHT

Day 6: Rejuvenation and Renewal as Your Healing Progresses

As you approach the final days of your healing journey, Day 6 offers an opportunity for rejuvenation and renewal as your body continues to respond to the healing interventions you've incorporated throughout the week. Dr. Barbara's holistic approach emphasizes the importance of nourishing your body, mind, and spirit with restorative practices that promote relaxation, vitality, and inner harmony.

Holistic Self-Care Practices

On Day 6, prioritize holistic self-care practices that nurture your body, mind, and spirit, fostering a sense of rejuvenation and renewal. Engage in activities that promote relaxation, stress reduction, and emotional well-being, such as meditation, deep breathing exercises, gentle movement, or spending time in nature. Allow yourself to fully immerse in these practices, letting go of any tension or worry and embracing the present moment with mindfulness and gratitude.

Dr. Barbara recommends incorporating self-care rituals that resonate with you personally and bring you joy and inner peace. This could include activities such as journaling, aromatherapy, listening to soothing music, or practicing creative expression through art or writing. Whatever practices you choose, prioritize activities that replenish your energy, restore your sense of balance, and nourish your soul.

Nourishing Meals and Hydration

Continue to nourish your body with wholesome, nutrient-dense meals and ample hydration on Day 6 to support your overall well-being and vitality. Enjoy a variety of colorful fruits and vegetables, whole grains, lean proteins, and healthy fats to provide your body with essential nutrients and antioxidants. Stay hydrated by drinking plenty of water throughout the day, supporting optimal cellular function and promoting detoxification and renewal.

Dr. Barbara recommends incorporating foods that are not only nourishing to the body but also satisfying to the soul. Prepare meals with love and intention, savoring each bite and appreciating the nourishment and vitality it provides. Take the time to sit down and enjoy your meals mindfully, paying attention to the flavors, textures, and sensations of the food, and expressing gratitude for the abundance of nourishment and healing it brings.

Connection and Community

As you reflect on your healing journey and the progress you've made on Day 6, seek connection and community to support and uplift you on your path. Reach out to friends, family members, or fellow participants to share your experiences, insights, and challenges, and to receive encouragement and support in return. Connection with others can be a source of strength and inspiration, reminding you that you are not alone on your healing journey.

Dr. Barbara encourages you to cultivate meaningful connections with others and to surround yourself with positive, supportive individuals who uplift and empower you. Share your journey openly and authentically, allowing yourself to be vulnerable and receiving the love and support that others have to offer. Together, you can celebrate your progress, acknowledge your achievements, and embrace the transformative power of healing and renewal.

Reflection and Gratitude

As Day 6 draws to a close, take time for reflection and gratitude, acknowledging the progress you've made on your healing journey and expressing appreciation for the support and resources that have guided you along the way. Reflect on the lessons you've learned, the challenges you've overcome, and the growth you've experienced, recognizing the resilience and strength within you.

Dr. Barbara encourages you to cultivate a spirit of gratitude for the abundance of blessings in your life, both big and small. Take a moment to express gratitude for your body's innate wisdom and healing capacity, for the love and support of friends and family, and for the opportunity to embark on this journey of self-discovery and transformation. With a heart full of gratitude and a spirit renewed, you can approach the final day of your healing journey with optimism, resilience, and a sense of empowerment.

Conclusion

Day 6 of your healing journey offers an opportunity for rejuvenation and renewal as you continue to nurture your body, mind, and spirit with restorative practices and nourishing self-care rituals. By prioritizing holistic self-care, nourishing meals, connection with others, and reflection and gratitude, you can support your body's natural healing processes and cultivate a sense of vitality, well-being, and inner harmony. With dedication, mindfulness, and a commitment to self-care, you can embrace the transformative power of healing and renewal as you approach the final day of your journey.

CHAPTER NINE

Day 7: Completing Your Cancer Cure and Transitioning to a Maintenance Plan

Congratulations on reaching the final day of your healing journey! Day 7 marks the culmination of your efforts and signifies a significant milestone in your path towards wellness. As you complete your cancer cure program, it's essential to reflect on your progress, celebrate your achievements, and transition to a maintenance plan that supports your long-term health and well-being. Dr. Barbara's holistic approach emphasizes the importance of integrating the lessons learned and habits developed during your healing journey into your daily life, empowering you to continue your journey towards optimal health and vitality.

Reflection and Celebration

Take time on Day 7 to reflect on your healing journey and celebrate the progress you've made. Acknowledge the challenges you've overcome, the insights you've gained, and the growth you've experienced along the way. Celebrate your resilience, determination, and commitment to your health and well-being, recognizing the transformational power of healing and self-discovery.

Dr. Barbara encourages you to express gratitude for the support and resources that have guided you on your journey, including the wisdom of nature, the expertise of healthcare providers, and the love and encouragement of friends and family. Celebrate your achievements with joy and gratitude, knowing that you have taken significant steps towards reclaiming your health and vitality.

Transition to a Maintenance Plan

As you complete your cancer cure program on Day 7, it's essential to transition to a maintenance plan that supports your long-term health and well-being. This plan may include ongoing lifestyle modifications, dietary changes, and self-care practices that promote resilience, vitality, and disease prevention. Dr. Barbara recommends incorporating the following elements into your maintenance plan:

1. **Healthy Nutrition**: Continue to prioritize a balanced diet rich in fruits, vegetables, whole grains, lean proteins, and healthy fats. Choose organic, locally sourced foods whenever possible, and minimize your intake of processed foods, sugary beverages, and artificial additives.

2. **Regular Exercise**: Maintain a regular exercise routine that includes a combination of aerobic exercise, strength training, and flexibility exercises. Aim for at least 150 minutes of moderate-intensity exercise or 75 minutes of vigorous-intensity exercise per week, as recommended by health guidelines.

3. **Stress Management**: Practice stress-reducing techniques such as meditation, deep breathing, yoga, tai chi, or progressive muscle relaxation to promote relaxation and emotional well-being. Prioritize activities that bring you joy, peace, and inner harmony, and make time for self-care rituals that nourish your body, mind, and spirit.

4. **Mindful Living**: Cultivate mindfulness and awareness in your daily life, paying attention to your thoughts, feelings, and sensations without judgment. Practice gratitude, compassion, and acceptance, embracing each moment with presence and openness.

5. **Regular Check-ups**: Schedule regular check-ups with your healthcare provider to monitor your health and well-being, including cancer screenings, blood tests, and other preventive measures. Stay informed about your health status and be proactive in addressing any concerns or symptoms that arise.

Continued Support and Community

As you transition to your maintenance plan on Day 7, remember that you are not alone on your journey towards wellness. Seek continued support from friends, family members, healthcare providers, and fellow participants who understand and support your commitment to health and vitality. Share your experiences, challenges, and successes with others, and draw strength and inspiration from the collective wisdom and encouragement of your community.

Dr. Barbara encourages you to stay connected with others who share your values and aspirations for optimal health and well-being. Join support groups, online forums, or community organizations dedicated to holistic health and wellness, and participate in events, workshops, or retreats that nourish your mind, body, and spirit. Together, you can continue to learn, grow, and thrive on your journey towards wholeness and vitality.

Conclusion

Day 7 of your healing journey marks the completion of your cancer cure program and the beginning of a new chapter in your path towards wellness. As you reflect on your progress, celebrate your achievements, and transition to a maintenance plan that supports your long-term health and vitality, know that you are empowered to continue your journey towards optimal health and well-being. With dedication, mindfulness, and a commitment to self-care, you can embrace the transformative power of healing and live a life of vitality, resilience, and joy.

CHAPTER TEN

Empowering Your Health: Integrating Dr. Barbara's Principles for Long-Term Wellness and Cancer Prevention

Dr. Barbara's holistic approach to health and wellness emphasizes the importance of empowering individuals to take an active role in their well-being, fostering resilience, vitality, and disease prevention. By integrating Dr. Barbara's principles for long-term wellness and cancer prevention into your daily life, you can cultivate a lifestyle that supports optimal health and vitality, empowering you to thrive in mind, body, and spirit.

1. Nourishing Nutrition

Prioritize a balanced diet rich in whole, nutrient-dense foods that provide essential vitamins, minerals, antioxidants, and phytonutrients to support optimal health and well-being. Emphasize fruits, vegetables, whole grains, lean proteins, and healthy fats, and minimize your intake of processed foods, sugary beverages, and artificial additives. Choose organic, locally sourced foods whenever possible, and aim to eat a rainbow of colors to ensure a diverse array of nutrients and phytochemicals.

2. Regular Physical Activity

Incorporate regular physical activity into your daily routine to promote cardiovascular health, muscular strength, flexibility, and overall well-being. Engage in a variety of activities that you enjoy, including aerobic exercise, strength training, yoga, Pilates, or recreational sports. Aim for at least 150 minutes of moderate-intensity exercise or 75 minutes of vigorous-intensity exercise per week, as recommended by health guidelines, and prioritize movement that brings you joy and vitality.

3. Stress Management

Practice stress-reducing techniques such as meditation, deep breathing, progressive muscle relaxation, or mindfulness to promote relaxation, emotional well-being, and resilience. Prioritize activities that help you unwind and recharge, such as spending time in nature, engaging in creative expression, or connecting with loved ones. Cultivate a positive mindset, and practice gratitude, optimism, and self-compassion to enhance your ability to cope with life's challenges and thrive in the face of adversity.

4. Mindful Living

Cultivate mindfulness and awareness in your daily life, paying attention to your thoughts, feelings, and sensations without judgment. Practice presence, acceptance, and non-reactivity, embracing each moment with openness and curiosity. Engage in activities that nourish your mind, body, and spirit, such as journaling, visualization, or spending time in quiet reflection.

Prioritize self-care and make time for activities that bring you joy, fulfillment, and inner peace.

5. Social Connection

Nurture meaningful connections with friends, family members, and community members who support and uplift you on your journey towards wellness. Share your experiences, challenges, and successes with others, and draw strength and inspiration from the collective wisdom and encouragement of your community. Join support groups, online forums, or community organizations dedicated to holistic health and wellness, and participate in events, workshops, or retreats that nourish your soul and deepen your sense of connection.

6. Preventive Healthcare

Take a proactive approach to your health by scheduling regular check-ups with your healthcare provider, including cancer screenings, blood tests, and other preventive measures. Stay informed about your health status and be proactive in addressing any concerns or symptoms that arise. Advocate for your health and well-being by asking questions, seeking second opinions, and taking an active role in decision-making regarding your healthcare.

7. Environmental Awareness

Be mindful of environmental factors that may impact your health and well-being, such as air and water quality, exposure to toxins and pollutants, and lifestyle habits. Take steps to minimize your exposure to harmful chemicals and pollutants by choosing organic, natural products whenever possible, and adopting eco-friendly practices that support environmental sustainability. Advocate for policies and initiatives that promote clean air, clean water, and a healthy environment for all.

By integrating Dr. Barbara's principles for long-term wellness and cancer prevention into your daily life, you can empower yourself to take control of your health and well-being, cultivate resilience, vitality, and disease prevention, and live a life of optimal health, vitality, and fulfillment. With dedication, mindfulness, and a commitment to holistic wellness, you can embrace the transformative power of healing and thrive in mind, body, and spirit.

Bio Ferro Tonic:

Definition: Bio Ferro Tonic is a dietary supplement primarily composed of herbs and minerals. It's often marketed as a natural way to support overall health, particularly by promoting blood health and circulation.

Ingredients: Typical ingredients in Bio Ferro Tonic may include a blend of herbs such as burdock root, yellow dock root, sarsaparilla root, and cascara sagrada bark, along with minerals like iron and potassium phosphate.

How to Prepare: Bio Ferro Tonic usually comes in liquid form and is typically taken orally. It's important to follow the instructions on the product label for dosage and administration.

Dosage: The dosage can vary depending on the specific product and individual needs. It's crucial to consult with a healthcare professional or follow the recommended dosage on the product label to avoid potential side effects.

How to Use: Bio Ferro Tonic is often taken by adding the recommended dosage to water or juice and consuming it orally. It's important to shake the bottle well before use and store it according to the manufacturer's instructions.

Side Effects: While Bio Ferro Tonic is generally considered safe when used as directed, some individuals may experience side effects such as digestive discomfort, allergic reactions, or interactions with medications. It's essential to consult with a healthcare provider before starting any new supplement regimen, especially if you have underlying health conditions or are taking medications.

Bladderwrack:

Definition: Bladderwrack is a type of seaweed or marine algae commonly used in traditional medicine and as a dietary supplement. It's known for its potential health benefits, particularly related to thyroid health and weight management.

Ingredients: Bladderwrack contains various nutrients, including iodine, vitamins, minerals, and antioxidants. The primary active components are iodine and fucoidan, a type of carbohydrate found in brown seaweeds.

How to Prepare: Bladderwrack supplements are available in various forms, including capsules, powders, and liquid extracts. They can be taken orally with water or added to smoothies and other beverages.

Dosage: The appropriate dosage of bladderwrack can vary based on factors such as age, health status, and the specific product being used. It's essential to follow the recommended dosage on the product label or consult with a healthcare professional for personalized guidance.

How to Use: Bladderwrack supplements are typically taken orally, either with water or mixed into food or beverages. It's important to follow the instructions on the product label and avoid exceeding the recommended dosage.

Side Effects: While bladderwrack is generally considered safe for most people when used in moderation, excessive intake of iodine from bladderwrack supplements can cause thyroid dysfunction and other adverse effects. Individuals with thyroid disorders, iodine sensitivity, or certain medical conditions should exercise caution and consult with a healthcare provider before using bladderwrack supplements. Common side effects may include digestive upset, allergic reactions, or interactions with medications.

Blood Purifier:

Definition: Blood purifiers are herbal remedies or dietary supplements believed to cleanse or detoxify the blood, often promoting overall health and well-being. They are thought to support the body's natural detoxification processes and improve blood circulation.

Ingredients: Blood purifiers may contain a variety of herbs and botanical extracts known for their purported cleansing and detoxifying properties. Common ingredients include burdock root, red clover, dandelion root, and yellow dock root, among others.

How to Prepare: Blood purifiers are typically available in various forms, including capsules, tablets, powders, and liquid extracts. They are usually taken orally with water or juice, following the recommended dosage on the product label.

Dosage: The dosage of blood purifiers can vary depending on the specific product and individual needs. It's important to adhere to the recommended dosage on the product label or consult with a healthcare professional for personalized guidance.

How to Use: Blood purifiers are typically taken orally, either with water or mixed into beverages. They are often used as part of a detoxification regimen or to support overall health and vitality.

Side Effects: While blood purifiers are generally considered safe for most people when used as directed, some individuals may experience side effects such as digestive discomfort, allergic reactions, or interactions with medications. It's important to consult with a healthcare provider before starting any new supplement regimen, especially if you have underlying health conditions or are taking medications.

Blue Vervain:

Definition: Blue vervain, also known as Verbena hastata, is a perennial herb native to North America. It has been used in traditional medicine for centuries to treat various ailments, including anxiety, insomnia, and digestive issues.

Ingredients: Blue vervain contains several active compounds, including aucubin, verbenalin, and volatile oils. These compounds are believed to contribute to the herb's medicinal properties.

How to Prepare: Blue vervain is typically consumed as a tea or tincture. To make tea, dried blue vervain leaves and flowers are steeped in hot water for several minutes before being strained and consumed. Tinctures are prepared by steeping the herb in alcohol or vinegar to extract its active compounds.

Dosage: The appropriate dosage of blue vervain can vary depending on factors such as age, health status, and the specific preparation being used. It's important to follow the recommended dosage on the product label or consult with a qualified herbalist or healthcare professional for personalized guidance.

How to Use: Blue vervain tea or tincture is typically taken orally. It can be consumed on its own or mixed with honey or other herbal teas for added flavor.

Side Effects: While blue vervain is generally considered safe for most people when used in moderation, excessive intake may cause digestive upset or allergic reactions in some individuals. Pregnant or breastfeeding women should avoid blue vervain due to its potential to stimulate uterine contractions. As with any herbal remedy, it's important to consult with a healthcare provider before using blue vervain, especially if you have underlying health conditions or are taking medications.

Bromide Plus Powder:

Definition: Bromide Plus Powder is a dietary supplement formulated to support thyroid health and promote overall well-being. It typically contains a blend of herbs and minerals that are believed to have beneficial effects on thyroid function.

Ingredients: Bromide Plus Powder often contains a combination of herbs such as bladderwrack, sea moss, and burdock root, along with minerals like iodine and potassium phosphate. These ingredients are thought to support thyroid function and maintain optimal iodine levels in the body.

How to Prepare: Bromide Plus Powder is usually mixed with water or juice to create a drinkable solution. It's important to follow the instructions on the product label for dosage and preparation.

Dosage: The dosage of Bromide Plus Powder can vary depending on the specific product and individual needs. It's crucial to consult with a healthcare professional or follow the recommended dosage on the product label to avoid potential side effects.

How to Use: Bromide Plus Powder is typically taken orally by mixing the recommended dosage with water or juice. It's important to shake or stir the mixture well before consuming it to ensure even distribution of the ingredients.

Side Effects: While Bromide Plus Powder is generally considered safe when used as directed, some individuals may experience side effects such as digestive discomfort or allergic reactions to certain ingredients. It's essential to consult with a healthcare provider before starting any new supplement regimen, especially if you have underlying health conditions or are taking medications.

Bugleweed:

Definition: Bugleweed, also known as Lycopusvirginicus, is a perennial herb native to North America and Europe. It has been used in traditional medicine to treat various conditions, including hyperthyroidism, anxiety, and insomnia.

Ingredients: Bugleweed contains several active compounds, including lithospermic acid, phenolic acids, and flavonoids. These compounds are believed to contribute to the herb's medicinal properties, particularly its ability to regulate thyroid function.

How to Prepare: Bugleweed is commonly consumed as a tea or tincture. To make tea, dried bugleweed leaves and flowers are steeped in hot water for several minutes before being strained and consumed. Tinctures are prepared by steeping the herb in alcohol or vinegar to extract its active compounds.

Dosage: The appropriate dosage of bugleweed can vary depending on factors such as age, health status, and the specific preparation being used. It's important to follow the recommended dosage on the product label or consult with a qualified herbalist or healthcare professional for personalized guidance.

How to Use: Bugleweed tea or tincture is typically taken orally. It can be consumed on its own or mixed with honey or other herbal teas for added flavor.

Side Effects: While bugleweed is generally considered safe for most people when used in moderation, excessive intake may cause digestive upset or allergic reactions in some individuals. Pregnant or breastfeeding women should avoid bugleweed due to its potential to stimulate uterine contractions. As with any herbal remedy, it's important to consult with a healthcare provider before using bugleweed, especially if you have underlying health conditions or are taking medications.

Burdock:

Definition: Burdock, scientifically known as Arctium lappa, is a biennial plant native to Europe and Asia but now found worldwide. It's part of the Asteraceae family and has been used for centuries in traditional medicine and culinary practices.

Ingredients: Burdock contains various nutrients, including carbohydrates, fiber, vitamins (such as vitamin B6, folate, and vitamin C), and minerals (including potassium, magnesium, and manganese). It also contains active compounds such as polyphenols and volatile oils.

How to Prepare: Burdock can be prepared and consumed in various ways. The roots, leaves, and seeds are all utilized for different purposes. The root is commonly used in cooking, herbal teas, tinctures, and supplements, while the leaves and seeds are sometimes used in herbal preparations.

Dosage: The appropriate dosage of burdock root can vary depending on the specific form and intended use. For culinary purposes, there are no strict dosage guidelines, but for supplements or herbal remedies, it's essential to follow the recommended dosage on the product label or consult with a healthcare professional.

How to Use: Burdock root can be used in cooking by peeling, slicing, and adding it to soups, stews, stir-fries, or salads. It can also be brewed into a tea or used to make tinctures or extracts for medicinal purposes. Some people may also take burdock root supplements in capsule or powder form.

Side Effects: While burdock is generally considered safe for most people when consumed in moderate amounts, some individuals may experience allergic reactions or digestive upset. Additionally, burdock may interact with certain medications or have adverse effects in individuals with certain health conditions, such as diabetes or allergies to plants in the Asteraceae family. It's important to consult with a healthcare provider before using burdock, especially if you have underlying health conditions or are taking medications.

Cascara Sagrada:

Definition: Cascara Sagrada, scientifically known as Rhamnus purshiana, is a species of buckthorn native to western North America. It has been used traditionally as a laxative and to promote bowel regularity.

Ingredients: The primary active ingredients in cascara sagrada are anthraquinone glycosides, particularly cascarosides A and B. These compounds stimulate peristalsis in the colon, leading to increased bowel movements.

How to Prepare: Cascara sagrada is typically prepared as an herbal tea, tincture, or capsule. To make tea, dried cascara sagrada bark is steeped in hot water for several minutes before being strained and consumed. Tinctures are prepared by steeping the bark in alcohol to extract its active compounds.

Dosage: The appropriate dosage of cascara sagrada can vary depending on the specific preparation and intended use. It's important to follow the recommended dosage on the product label or consult with a healthcare professional for personalized guidance.

How to Use: Cascara sagrada tea or tincture is typically taken orally. It's important to start with a low dose and gradually increase if needed to avoid potential side effects such as cramping or diarrhea.

Side Effects: Cascara sagrada is considered safe for short-term use when used as directed. However, long-term or excessive use may lead to dependence, electrolyte imbalance, or dehydration. It may also interact with certain medications or have adverse effects in individuals with certain health conditions. It's important to use cascara sagrada under the guidance of a healthcare professional and to discontinue use if any adverse effects occur.

Cell Food:

Definition: Cell Food is a dietary supplement marketed as a highly oxygenating and alkalizing formula. It's claimed to support overall health and vitality by providing essential nutrients and oxygen to the cells.

Ingredients: The exact ingredients of Cell Food can vary depending on the brand, but it typically contains a proprietary blend of minerals, enzymes, electrolytes, and trace elements. Some common ingredients may include purified water, dissolved oxygen, seawater extract, and plant-based enzymes.

How to Prepare: Cell Food is usually available in liquid form and is typically taken orally. It can be consumed directly or diluted in water or juice before consumption.

Dosage: The dosage of Cell Food can vary depending on the specific product and individual needs. It's important to follow the recommended dosage on the product label or consult with a healthcare professional for personalized guidance.

How to Use: Cell Food is typically taken orally, either directly or mixed into water or juice. It's important to shake the bottle well before use and to store it according to the manufacturer's instructions.

Side Effects: Cell Food is generally considered safe for most people when used as directed. However, some individuals may experience mild digestive upset or allergic reactions to certain ingredients. It's essential to consult with a healthcare provider before starting any new supplement regimen, especially if you have underlying health conditions or are taking medications.

Chaparral:

Definition: Chaparral, scientifically known as Larrea tridentata, is a shrub native to the southwestern United States and northern Mexico. It has been used for centuries by Native American tribes for its medicinal properties and is commonly used in herbal medicine today.

Ingredients: Chaparral contains several bioactive compounds, including nordihydroguaiaretic acid (NDGA), flavonoids, lignans, and volatile oils. NDGA is believed to be the primary active compound responsible for many of chaparral's therapeutic effects.

How to Prepare: Chaparral can be prepared and consumed in various forms, including teas, tinctures, capsules, and topical preparations. To make tea, dried chaparral leaves are steeped in hot water for several minutes before being strained and consumed. Tinctures are prepared by steeping the herb in alcohol or vinegar to extract its active compounds.

Dosage: The appropriate dosage of chaparral can vary depending on the specific form and intended use. It's important to follow the recommended dosage on the product label or consult with a healthcare professional for personalized guidance.

How to Use: Chaparral tea or tincture is typically taken orally. It can also be applied topically to the skin for certain conditions. It's important to use chaparral products as directed and to discontinue use if any adverse effects occur.

Side Effects: Chaparral is generally considered safe for most people when used in moderate amounts. However, excessive intake or prolonged use may lead to liver toxicity or other adverse effects. It may also interact with certain medications or have adverse effects in individuals with certain health conditions. It's important to use chaparral under the guidance of a healthcare professional and to discontinue use if any adverse effects occur.

Cocolmeca:

Definition: Cocolmeca, also known as Smilax ornata or sarsaparilla, is a flowering vine native to Mexico and Central America. It has been used traditionally in Mexican and Central American folk medicine for its purported medicinal properties.

Ingredients: Cocolmeca contains various bioactive compounds, including saponins, flavonoids, and plant sterols. These compounds are believed to contribute to the herb's medicinal properties, including its potential as a diuretic, blood purifier, and anti-inflammatory agent.

How to Prepare: Cocolmeca is commonly prepared and consumed as an herbal tea or decoction. To make tea, dried cocolmeca roots or leaves are steeped in hot water for several minutes before being strained and consumed. Decoctions involve boiling the roots or leaves in water to extract their active compounds.

Dosage: The appropriate dosage of cocolmeca can vary depending on factors such as age, health status, and the specific preparation being used. It's important to follow the recommended dosage on the product label or consult with a qualified herbalist or healthcare professional for personalized guidance.

How to Use: Cocolmeca tea or decoction is typically taken orally. It can also be used topically for certain skin conditions. It's important to use cocolmeca products as directed and to discontinue use if any adverse effects occur.

Side Effects: Cocolmeca is generally considered safe for most people when used in moderate amounts. However, excessive intake may lead to digestive upset or other adverse effects. It may also interact with certain medications or have adverse effects in individuals with certain health conditions. It's important to use cocolmeca under the guidance of a healthcare professional and to discontinue use if any adverse effects occur.

Guaco:

Definition: Guaco, also known as Mikania cordata or Mikania glomerata, is a medicinal plant native to Central and South America. It has a long history of use in traditional medicine for its potential therapeutic properties.

Ingredients: Guaco contains several bioactive compounds, including coumarins, flavonoids, tannins, and saponins. These compounds are believed to contribute to the herb's medicinal properties, including its potential as an expectorant, anti-inflammatory, and antispasmodic agent.

How to Prepare: Guaco is typically prepared and consumed as an herbal tea or infusion. To make tea, dried guaco leaves are steeped in hot water for several minutes before being strained and consumed.

Dosage: The appropriate dosage of guaco can vary depending on factors such as age, health status, and the specific preparation being used. It's important to follow the recommended dosage on the product label or consult with a qualified herbalist or healthcare professional for personalized guidance.

How to Use: Guaco tea is typically taken orally. It can be consumed on its own or mixed with honey or other herbal teas for added flavor.

Side Effects: Guaco is generally considered safe for most people when used in moderate amounts. However, some individuals may experience allergic reactions or digestive upset. It may also interact with certain medications or have adverse effects in individuals with certain health conditions. It's important to use guaco under the guidance of a healthcare professional and to discontinue use if any adverse effects occur.

Herban Iron:

Definition: Herban Iron is a dietary supplement designed to provide an easily absorbable form of iron to support healthy iron levels in the body. It's particularly beneficial for individuals with iron deficiency or anemia.

Ingredients: Herban Iron typically contains iron in the form of ferrous bisglycinate, which is a highly bioavailable and gentle form of iron that is less likely to cause digestive upset or constipation compared to other forms of iron. It may also contain other ingredients such as vitamin C to enhance iron absorption.

How to Prepare: Herban Iron is usually available in capsule or liquid form. Capsules are taken orally with water, while liquid forms may be mixed with water or juice before consumption. It's important to follow the recommended dosage on the product label.

Dosage: The appropriate dosage of Herban Iron depends on factors such as age, gender, and the severity of iron deficiency. It's important to consult with a healthcare professional to determine the correct dosage for individual needs.

How to Use: Herban Iron capsules are typically taken orally with water, while liquid forms may be mixed with water or juice before consumption. It's important to take Herban Iron as directed and to avoid taking it with dairy products, antacids, or other substances that may interfere with iron absorption.

Side Effects: While Herban Iron is generally considered safe for most people when used as directed, some individuals may experience mild side effects such as gastrointestinal discomfort or constipation. It's important to consult with a healthcare professional before starting any new supplement regimen, especially if you have underlying health conditions or are taking medications.

Hydrangea:

Definition: Hydrangea, scientifically known as Hydrangea arborescens, is a flowering shrub native to North America. It has been used traditionally in herbal medicine for its potential diuretic and anti-inflammatory properties.

Ingredients: Hydrangea contains several bioactive compounds, including saponins, flavonoids, and glycosides. These compounds are believed to contribute to the herb's medicinal properties, including its potential as a diuretic, kidney tonic, and anti-inflammatory agent.

How to Prepare: Hydrangea root is typically prepared and consumed as an herbal tea or tincture. To make tea, dried hydrangea root is steeped in hot water for several minutes before being strained and consumed. Tinctures are prepared by steeping the root in alcohol or vinegar to extract its active compounds.

Dosage: The appropriate dosage of hydrangea can vary depending on factors such as age, health status, and the specific preparation being used. It's important to follow the recommended dosage on the product label or consult with a qualified herbalist or healthcare professional for personalized guidance.

How to Use: Hydrangea tea or tincture is typically taken orally. It's important to use hydrangea products as directed and to discontinue use if any adverse effects occur.

Side Effects: Hydrangea is generally considered safe for most people when used in moderate amounts. However, some individuals may experience digestive upset or allergic reactions. It may also interact with certain medications or have adverse effects in individuals with certain health conditions. It's important to use hydrangea under the guidance of a healthcare professional and to discontinue use if any adverse effects occur.

Irish Moss:

Definition: Irish Moss, scientifically known as Chondrus crispus, is a species of red algae or seaweed native to the Atlantic coastlines of Europe and North America. It has been used for centuries in traditional Irish and Scottish cuisine, as well as in herbal medicine.

Ingredients: Irish Moss is rich in various nutrients, including iodine, sulfur compounds, vitamins (such as vitamin A, vitamin K, and vitamin B12), minerals (including calcium, magnesium, potassium, and sodium), and polysaccharides (such as carrageenan). These nutrients are believed to contribute to the herb's potential health benefits.

How to Prepare: Irish Moss is typically prepared by soaking it in water to rehydrate and soften it before use. It can be added to soups, stews, smoothies, desserts, and other dishes as a thickening agent or nutritional supplement.

Dosage: The appropriate dosage of Irish Moss can vary depending on factors such as age, health status, and the specific preparation being used. It's important to follow recipes or guidelines for culinary use and to consult with a healthcare professional for guidance on using Irish Moss as a dietary supplement.

How to Use: Irish Moss can be used in culinary applications to add thickness and nutritional value to dishes. It can also be consumed as a dietary supplement in the form of capsules, powders, or extracts.

Side Effects: Irish Moss is generally considered safe for most people when consumed in moderate amounts as part of a balanced diet. However, some individuals may be allergic to seaweed or carrageenan, a compound found in Irish Moss that is used as a food additive. It's important to discontinue use if any adverse effects occur and to consult with a healthcare professional if you have any concerns.

Red Clover:

Definition: Red clover, scientifically known as Trifolium pratense, is a flowering plant belonging to the legume family. It's native to Europe, Western Asia, and Northwest Africa but has been naturalized in many other regions. Red clover has been used in traditional medicine for various purposes, including its potential to support women's health and menopausal symptoms.

Ingredients: Red clover contains several bioactive compounds, including isoflavones (such as genistein and daidzein), flavonoids, and phytoestrogens. These compounds are believed to contribute to the herb's medicinal properties, including its potential as a hormone-balancing agent and its ability to support cardiovascular health.

How to Prepare: Red clover is typically prepared and consumed as an herbal tea or tincture. To make tea, dried red clover flowers are steeped in hot water for several minutes before being strained and consumed. Tinctures are prepared by steeping the flowers in alcohol or vinegar to extract their active compounds.

Dosage: The appropriate dosage of red clover can vary depending on factors such as age, health status, and the specific preparation being used. It's important to follow the recommended dosage on the product label or consult with a qualified herbalist or healthcare professional for personalized guidance.

How to Use: Red clover tea or tincture is typically taken orally. It's important to use red clover products as directed and to discontinue use if any adverse effects occur.

Side Effects: Red clover is generally considered safe for most people when used in moderate amounts. However, some individuals may experience allergic reactions or digestive upset. It may also interact with certain medications or have adverse effects in individuals with certain health conditions. It's important to use red clover under the guidance of a healthcare professional and to discontinue use if any adverse effects occur.

Red Raspberry:

Definition: Red raspberry, scientifically known as Rubus idaeus, is a species of raspberry native to Europe and northern Asia. It's widely cultivated for its delicious berries and has been used in traditional medicine for various purposes, including its potential to support women's health during pregnancy and childbirth.

Ingredients: Red raspberry contains several bioactive compounds, including flavonoids, ellagic acid, anthocyanins, and vitamin C. These compounds are believed to contribute to the herb's medicinal properties, including its potential as an antioxidant, anti-inflammatory, and uterine tonic.

How to Prepare: Red raspberry leaf is typically prepared and consumed as an herbal tea or infusion. To make tea, dried red raspberry leaves are steeped in hot water for several minutes before being strained and consumed.

Dosage: The appropriate dosage of red raspberry leaf can vary depending on factors such as age, health status, and the specific preparation being used. It's important to follow the recommended dosage on the product label or consult with a qualified herbalist or healthcare professional for personalized guidance.

How to Use: Red raspberry leaf tea is typically taken orally. It's often recommended for pregnant individuals in the later stages of pregnancy to support uterine health and prepare for childbirth. It's important to use red raspberry leaf products as directed and to discontinue use if any adverse effects occur.

Side Effects: Red raspberry leaf is generally considered safe for most people when used in moderate amounts. However, some individuals may experience allergic reactions or digestive upset. Pregnant individuals should consult with a healthcare professional before using red raspberry leaf, especially if they have any underlying health conditions or are taking medications. It's important to use red raspberry leaf under the guidance of a healthcare professional and to discontinue use if any adverse effects occur.

Rhubarb:

Definition: Rhubarb, scientifically known as Rheum rhabarbarum, is a perennial plant cultivated for its edible stalks. While primarily used in culinary applications, rhubarb has also been utilized in traditional medicine for its potential health benefits, particularly for digestive health.

Ingredients: Rhubarb stalks contain various bioactive compounds, including anthraquinones (such as emodin and rhein), fiber, vitamins (such as vitamin K), and minerals (including calcium and potassium). These compounds are believed to contribute to the herb's medicinal properties, including its potential as a laxative and digestive aid.

How to Prepare: Rhubarb stalks are typically cooked before consumption, as the raw stalks are very tart and can be unpleasant to eat. They are often used in pies, crisps, jams, sauces, and other desserts, as well as in savory dishes. Rhubarb can also be used to make compotes, jams, and preserves.

Dosage: There is no specific dosage for rhubarb in culinary applications, as it is used as a food rather than a medicinal herb. However, when used for its potential laxative effects, it's important to consume rhubarb in moderation to avoid gastrointestinal upset.

How to Use: Rhubarb stalks can be chopped and cooked in various dishes, including pies, sauces, and jams. It's important to remove and discard the leaves, as they contain toxic compounds. When using rhubarb for its potential laxative effects, it's typically consumed as part of a cooked dish or in the form of a rhubarb-based herbal remedy.

Side Effects: Rhubarb stalks are generally safe for most people when consumed in moderate amounts as part of a balanced diet.

However, excessive intake may lead to digestive upset or adverse effects due to the presence of oxalic acid, which can bind to calcium and form kidney stones in susceptible individuals. It's important to use rhubarb in moderation and to consult with a healthcare professional if you have any concerns or underlying health conditions.**Irish Sea Moss:**

Definition: Irish Sea Moss is a term often used interchangeably with Irish Moss, referring to the same species of red algae, Chondrus crispus. It's harvested from the rocky shores of the Atlantic coastlines of Europe and North America.

Ingredients: Irish Sea Moss shares the same nutritional profile as Irish Moss, containing iodine, vitamins, minerals, and polysaccharides. It's valued for its potential health benefits, including supporting thyroid function, boosting immune health, and promoting digestion.

How to Prepare: Irish Sea Moss is prepared in the same way as Irish Moss, by soaking it in water to rehydrate and soften it before use. It can be used in culinary applications or consumed as a dietary supplement.

Dosage: The dosage of Irish Sea Moss depends on the form and intended use. As a dietary supplement, it's important to follow the recommended dosage on the product label or consult with a healthcare professional for personalized guidance.

How to Use: Irish Sea Moss can be used in various culinary applications, including soups, smoothies, desserts, and sauces. It can also be consumed as a dietary supplement in the form of capsules, powders, or extracts.

Side Effects: Similar to Irish Moss, Irish Sea Moss is generally considered safe for most people when consumed in moderate amounts. However, individuals with seaweed allergies or sensitivities to carrageenan should exercise caution. It's important to discontinue use if any adverse effects occur and to consult with a healthcare professional if you have any concerns.

Lymphalin:

Definition: Lymphalin is a herbal supplement formulated to support lymphatic system health. The lymphatic system plays a crucial role in immune function and waste removal in the body, and Lymphalin is designed to promote its proper function.

Ingredients: Lymphalin typically contains a blend of herbs and botanical extracts known for their traditional use in supporting lymphatic system health. Common ingredients may include cleavers, red clover, echinacea, burdock root, and calendula, among others.

How to Prepare: Lymphalin is usually available in capsule or liquid form. Capsules are taken orally with water, while liquid forms may be mixed with water or juice before consumption. It's important to follow the recommended dosage on the product label.

Dosage: The appropriate dosage of Lymphalin can vary depending on the specific product and individual needs. It's important to follow the recommended dosage on the product label or consult with a healthcare professional for personalized guidance.

How to Use: Lymphalin capsules are typically taken orally with water, while liquid forms may be mixed with water or juice before consumption. It's often recommended to take Lymphalin on an empty stomach for optimal absorption.

Side Effects: Lymphalin is generally considered safe for most people when used as directed. However, some individuals may experience mild side effects such as gastrointestinal discomfort or allergic reactions to certain ingredients. It's important to consult with a healthcare provider before starting any new supplement regimen, especially if you have underlying health conditions or are taking medications.

Manjakani:

Definition: Manjakani, also known as Quercus infectoria or oak gall, is a natural substance derived from the oak tree. It has been used for centuries in traditional medicine for its potential health benefits, particularly for women's health and vaginal tightening.

Ingredients: Manjakani contains various bioactive compounds, including tannins, flavonoids, and gallic acid. These compounds are believed to contribute to the herb's medicinal properties, including its potential as an astringent and antiseptic agent.

How to Prepare: Manjakani is typically available in powder, capsule, or liquid extract form. It can be taken orally or used topically depending on the intended use. For vaginal tightening, manjakani may be applied topically as a gel or inserted into the vagina in capsule form.

Dosage: The appropriate dosage of manjakani can vary depending on factors such as age, health status, and the specific preparation being used. It's important to follow the recommended dosage on the product label or consult with a qualified herbalist or healthcare professional for personalized guidance.

How to Use: Manjakani can be taken orally or used topically depending on the intended use. It's important to use manjakani products as directed and to discontinue use if any adverse effects occur.

Side Effects: Manjakani is generally considered safe for most people when used in moderate amounts. However, some individuals may experience allergic reactions or skin irritation when used topically. It's important to use manjakani under the guidance of a healthcare professional and to discontinue use if any adverse effects occur.

Contribo:

Definition: Contribo, also known as Aristolochiatrilobata, is a vine native to the Caribbean and Central America. It has been used traditionally in folk medicine for various purposes, including as a remedy for digestive issues, inflammation, and pain relief.

Ingredients: Contribo contains several bioactive compounds, including aristolochic acids, flavonoids, and alkaloids. These compounds are believed to contribute to the herb's medicinal properties, including its potential as an anti-inflammatory and analgesic agent.

How to Prepare: Contribo is typically prepared and consumed as an herbal tea or decoction. To make tea, dried contribo leaves or stems are steeped in hot water for several minutes before being strained and consumed. Decoctions involve boiling the leaves or stems in water to extract their active compounds.

Dosage: The appropriate dosage of contribo can vary depending on factors such as age, health status, and the specific preparation being used. It's important to follow the recommended dosage on the product label or consult with a qualified herbalist or healthcare professional for personalized guidance.

How to Use: Contribo tea or decoction is typically taken orally. It's important to use contribo products as directed and to discontinue use if any adverse effects occur.

Side Effects: Contribo contains aristolochic acids, which have been associated with serious adverse effects, including kidney damage and cancer. Due to these safety concerns, the use of contribo is highly discouraged, and it's important to avoid products containing aristolochic acids. Individuals should seek alternative remedies for their health needs.

Dandelion Root:

Definition: Dandelion, scientifically known as Taraxacum officinale, is a common flowering plant found worldwide. While often considered a pesky weed, dandelion has a long history of use in traditional medicine for its various health benefits.

Ingredients: Dandelion root contains several bioactive compounds, including sesquiterpene lactones, triterpenes, flavonoids, and polysaccharides. These compounds are believed to contribute to the herb's medicinal properties, including its potential as a diuretic, digestive aid, and liver tonic.

How to Prepare: Dandelion root can be prepared and consumed in various forms, including teas, tinctures, capsules, and extracts. To make tea, dried dandelion root is steeped in hot water for several minutes before being strained and consumed. Tinctures are prepared by steeping the root in alcohol or vinegar to extract its active compounds.

Dosage: The appropriate dosage of dandelion root can vary depending on factors such as age, health status, and the specific preparation being used. It's important to follow the recommended dosage on the product label or consult with a qualified herbalist or healthcare professional for personalized guidance.

How to Use: Dandelion root tea, tincture, or capsules are typically taken orally. It's important to use dandelion root products as directed and to discontinue use if any adverse effects occur.

Side Effects: Dandelion root is generally considered safe for most people when used in moderate amounts. However, some individuals may experience allergic reactions or digestive upset. It may also interact with certain medications or have adverse effects in individuals with certain health conditions. It's important to use dandelion root under the guidance of a healthcare professional and to discontinue use if any adverse effects occur.

Green Food Plus:

Definition: Green Food Plus is a dietary supplement formulated to provide a concentrated source of nutrients derived from various green plants. It's designed to support overall health and well-being by delivering essential vitamins, minerals, antioxidants, and phytonutrients.

Ingredients: Green Food Plus typically contains a blend of powdered green vegetables, grasses, algae, and other plant-based ingredients. Common ingredients may include wheatgrass, barley grass, spirulina, chlorella, alfalfa, kale, spinach, and broccoli, among others.

How to Prepare: Green Food Plus is usually available in powder form and can be mixed with water, juice, or smoothies. It's important to follow the recommended dosage on the product label and to consume it as part of a balanced diet.

Dosage: The appropriate dosage of Green Food Plus can vary depending on the specific product and individual needs. It's important to follow the recommended dosage on the product label or consult with a healthcare professional for personalized guidance.

How to Use: Green Food Plus powder is typically mixed with water, juice, or smoothies and consumed orally. It's often taken once or twice daily, preferably with meals, to maximize nutrient absorption.

Side Effects: Green Food Plus is generally considered safe for most people when used as directed. However, some individuals may experience digestive upset or allergic reactions to certain ingredients. It's important to consult with a healthcare provider before starting any new supplement regimen, especially if you have underlying health conditions or are taking medications.

THE END

www.ingramcontent.com/pod-product-compliance
Lightning Source LLC
Chambersburg PA
CBHW081558250726
48653CB00009B/3496